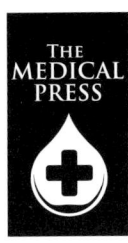

The Pocket Guide to Stayin' Alive

How to live a longer and healthier life

Peter Altman

THE MEDICAL PRESS

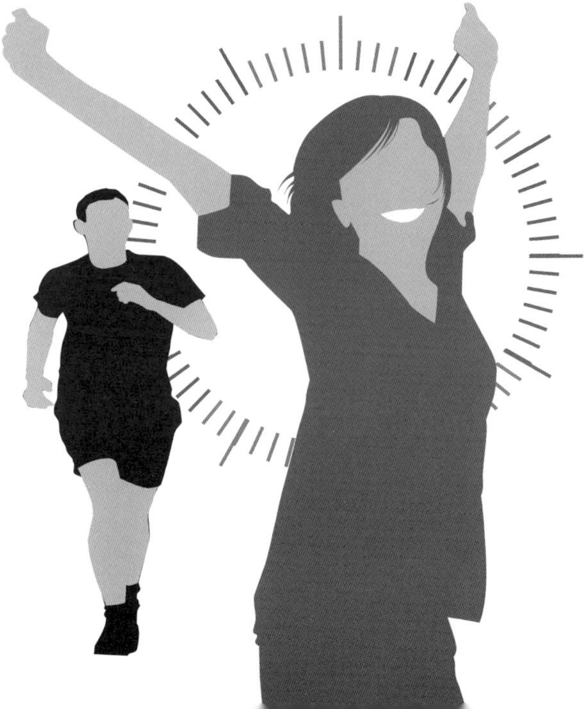

Published by The Medical Press
7 Ash Copse, Bricket Wood, St Albans AL2 3YA, UK

First edition 2010
Copyright © The Medical Press

ISBN 978 09557582 1 8
info@themedicalpress.co.uk

The publisher makes no representation, express or implied, with regard to the accuracy of the information in this book, and does not accept any legal responsibility or liability for any errors or omissions that may be made. The information is given in good faith, but is for guidance only, and patients should always discuss treatment options with their own Health Care Team.

CONTENTS

Foreword	1
Preface	3
CHAPTER 1 Losing weight	7
CHAPTER 2 Blood pressure	17
CHAPTER 3 Cholesterol	25
CHAPTER 4 Stroke	31
CHAPTER 5 Diabetes	37
CHAPTER 6 Cancer	45
CHAPTER 7 Will I have a heart attack?	55
CHAPTER 8 Eye tests	61
CHAPTER 9 Lung function tests	63
CHAPTER 10 Your own MOT (Medical & Optical Test) check list	65
CHAPTER 11 Vitamins and supplements	67
CHAPTER 12 Some medical myths	73
CHAPTER 13 Glossary	75
CHAPTER 14 A few last words	81
CHAPTER 15 Appendix	83
Index	87

Foreword

I'm delighted to report that first impressions are often wrong, and mine are no exception. My first reaction as I scanned through this book was 'not another self help book – this is all common sense'. But that is the whole point. It is all common sense, which is precisely what so many sources of information for the public don't offer. This book doesn't promise miracle cures or quick fixes; it doesn't pretend to have all the answers. But it does give you all the facts without the flannel, and lets you make up your own mind what to do with them.

This book is practical, comprehensive, but above all readable. Each section is neatly punctuated with checklists and for the mechanically minded (heaven forbid I should suggest that means the blokes) there are just enough MOT analogies to make you feel at home. Want to get healthier one step at a time? This book is a good place to start.

Dr Sarah Jarvis MA BM BCh DRCOG FRCGP

Preface

No-one likes being ill. It's a good idea therefore to look after ourselves so that our chances of getting ill are as low as possible. For example, if you are on a crowded train and another passenger is coughing and sneezing, it would make sense to stay as far away from him or her as possible, so that you have less chance of catching their germs. Or, if you want to cross a busy road, it makes sense to be very careful so that you don't get run over.

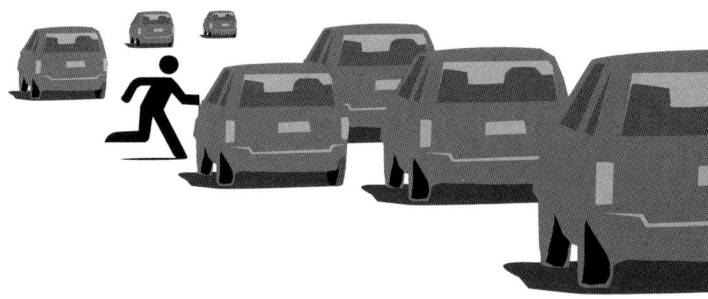

You probably learned how to cross a road, and to stay away from people who were coughing and sneezing, when you were quite young. These are things that we learn at school, or from our parents, and we remember them for the rest of our lives.

These are two very obvious things that most people would do. However, there are lots of other things that we can do to look after ourselves that will also lower our chances of getting ill and even increase our chances of living longer. It's no secret – don't get overweight, don't smoke, do take regular exercise, and do have regular medical check-ups.

Your body is a wonderful creation that can carry on doing its job for very many years. The oldest person who ever lived, with proper documents to prove it, was a French lady called Jeanne Calment. She was born in 1875 and died, aged 122 years and 164 days, in 1997. Of course, that was exceptional, and most people don't expect to live that long; to stay healthy and make it into your 80s or 90s is probably a good result. Your body can do it, but it does need some help along the way.

Think of a car. The engine was built to last for at least 100,000 miles, but it has lots of moving parts so needs looking after. It needs regular oil, battery and tyre pressure checks, among other things. In the same way, your body needs to be looked after to make sure that it is running properly.

Most bodies fail due to diseases of the heart and circulation (heart attacks, stroke), diabetes, lung disease, and cancer. Of course, everyone has to die eventually, but let's try and make it later rather than sooner. Let's try Stayin' Alive a bit longer.

That's what this book is about. It's a sort of check list of important items that you need to be aware of, and to make sure that they are all running properly. Just like a garage will go through a check list of items when your car goes in for its MOT test, so this book will take you through your own check list to see if your body has passed its own test. If it hasn't, there will be some advice on how to pass next time.

The first few chapters deal with weight and weight loss, blood pressure, cholesterol, and diabetes. These are sometimes called risk factors. A risk factor is something that can increase the chances of an event happening. For example, getting sun burnt is a risk factor for skin cancer. Being overweight, having too high a blood pressure and total cholesterol, having diabetes, and being a smoker, are all risk factors for heart attacks and strokes. Not looking out for traffic when you're crossing a busy road is a risk factor for getting run over.

A recurring theme in the book is a focus on numbers, such as waist measurement, blood pressure, cholesterol etc. Studies on hundreds of thousands of people around the World have shown in what range these numbers should be for optimum health. It's also been found that due to genetic reasons (that is, due to things that have been inherited from parents), some ethnic groups are at a higher risk so that their numbers will be different. This is especially true for people of Asian and African Caribbean origins.

Nowadays, doctors tend to look at a patient's total list of risk factors, so although it is obviously a good thing to have a normal blood pressure, this needs to be seen in conjunction with all the other risk factors. Think of it as a package – you wouldn't buy a hamper of fruit and vegetables if only the apples and carrots were in good condition.

Finally, smoking. This is a dreadful habit that is a serious risk factor for heart disease, strokes, diabetes, and lung disease including cancer. It is of course very easy for a non-smoker to tell someone else to stop smoking. The addiction to nicotine is hard to break, and even the prospect of better future health isn't always persuasive enough. There is help though. Various therapies and several new drug treatments can be very effective. Even though you may have smoked for many years, there will be an immediate health (and financial) benefit from stopping. If these words don't help, look at the drawings in the Smoking section on page 53.

1 Losing weight

Losing weight is a very popular pastime. Google has over 200 million entries for the word diet, and Amazon lists over 35,000 books with the word diet in the title. You'd think that with all this advice, someone would have come up with a perfect solution.

Unfortunately, as we all know, there is no easy answer to this problem. Although losing weight is easy in theory – just eat less and exercise more – it is very hard in practice. The main reason is that the foods that taste the best are often the ones that contain lots of fat and sugar, and it's the fat and sugar that makes us overweight. Think of french fries, cakes, chocolate, sweets, burgers. McDonald's has sold more than 100 billion (100,000,000,000) hamburgers, and continues to sell them at a rate of more than 6 million every day. Do they taste good? Yes, especially with a portion of french fries. Will they make you fat? Yes. Is this bad for your health? Yes.

The first thing we need to do is to see if we are, in fact, overweight. Various methods have been used for working this out, but now most health care teams use a very simple method that you can do yourself at home. It's your waist measurement and all you need is a tape measure.

It's very important to realize that your waist measurement may not be the same as your trouser measurement. Many overweight people will wear their trousers below their belly, as shown in the diagram on page 8. In this case, the trouser size is NOT the same as the waist size.

A proper waist measurement is taken as follows

- Place a tape measure to pass over your belly button and make sure that it is parallel to the ground
- Hold the tape snugly but not pressing into the skin
- Breathe out and take the reading

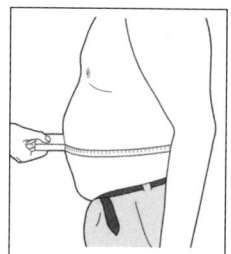

So, now it's time for our first Check List.

Check list 1	Waist Measurement
Ethnicity	Maximum desirable waist measurement
White male	102cm - 40in
White female	88cm - 34.5 in
Asian/African Caribbean male	90cm - 35.5 in
Asian/African Caribbean female	80cm - 31.5 in

Figures are given for men and women, and also for white people and for those who are Asian or Black African Caribbean. The numbers are given in inches and in centimeters for normal healthy people. They are the maximum desirable figures and are not targets – less would be better. If you have diabetes, or have or have had any form of heart disease, then your figures should definitely be lower.

You may be surprised that your height is not taken into account. This is because what is important is not so much your weight but where it is distributed on your body. It's more dangerous to your health to have extra fat around your middle than around your thighs.

Have you passed? If so, then well done. You're probably not overweight but if your waist measurement is close to the limit, then it wouldn't hurt to lose some weight and get it even lower.

But what if you failed? First, this means that you are almost certainly overweight, which you probably knew already. More importantly though, it means that your health could be at risk. You are more likely to have an increased risk of having a heart attack, a stroke, and developing diabetes. If that worries you, then good, because you have already taken the first step.

You may also come across another measure that is used to see if someone is overweight, and this is the BODY MASS INDEX (BMI). The BMI is calculated from your weight and your height. Measurements taken from many thousands of people have led to the conclusion that a healthy BMI should be between 20 and 25 for a man, and 19 and 24 for a women. If you're of Asian or Black African Caribbean descent, then your limits will be slightly lower. See the Glossary for an explanation of how the BMI is calculated.

To save making these calculations, here is a chart so that you can read off your height and weight, and then see the result on the chart. The ideal result would be in the pale pink region.

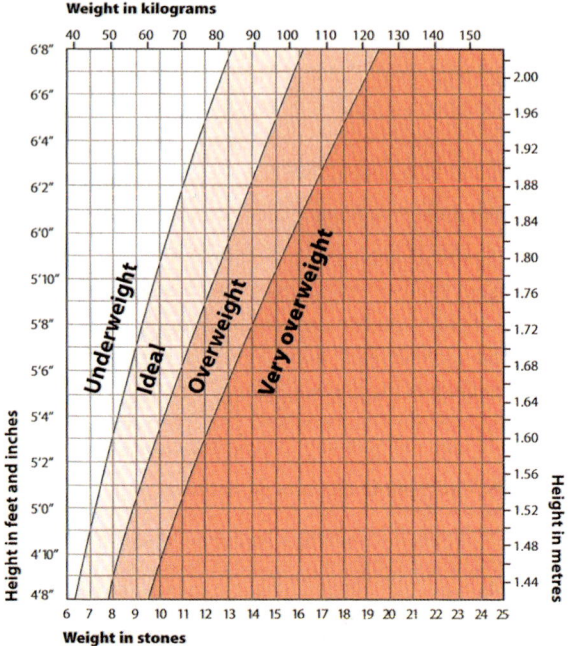

Chart for calculating whether or not you are overweight (adapted by the Food Standards Agency from a chart originally published by the British Heart Foundation, and reproduced with their kind permission)

So here is our second check list. These figures are for men – women will be about 1 less for each number. For example, a normal BMI result for a white woman would be 19 to 24.

Check list 2	Body Mass Index	
	White Men	Asian or African Caribbean Men
underweight	less than 20	less than 19
normal weight	20 to 25	19 to 23
overweight	25 to 30	23 to 27
obese	30 to 40	27 to 40
very obese	over 40	over 40

If you're in the obese or very obese range, then your weight is a serious health risk and you must get urgent professional help to reduce it.

The easiest way to approach the problem of losing weight is to have a strong motivation, and what better motivation than being able to increase your chances of having a long and healthy life? To start with, it may be helpful to explain a little about energy, calories, and weight, and how they are related.

Calories and energy

Without going into lots of detail, the body needs a supply of energy to keep it going, much like a car needs a supply of fuel to keep it going. The food we eat gets turned into energy by the body, which is then used up in our daily activities. This energy is measured in units called calories. One thousand calories is called a kilocalorie (kcal) and it is these units that are commonly used on food packaging and in weight-loss charts etc. You will also see units called kiloJoules - kJ. These are metric equivalents that we are all supposed to be using. One kilocalorie equals just over 4 kiloJoules.

Obviously, someone who sits in an office all day will use up far less energy (kilocalories) than someone who is chopping wood all day. Doctors and scientists have worked out approximately how many kilocalories are used up in various occupations and activities.

Here are some of the results; the numbers are kilocalories used per hour. They are only a guide, since the exact figures will depend on various things, including your age, weight, and sex.

75	200	400	800
reading	walking	jogging	squash
driving	cleaning	football	running up stairs
sleeping	painting	swimming	chopping wood
watching TV		tennis	
office work			

It's easy to work out that if you spend your day with 8 hours in an office, 8 hours in bed, 4 hours watching TV, and the remaining 4 hours reading and driving, then you'll use up 75 times 24 which equals 1,800 kilocalories per day.

On the other hand, if you're an active sportsperson and you have a heavy manual day job, you could easily use up several thousand kilocalories in a day.

Most people would fit in somewhere between, needing about 2,000 (for women) and 2,500 (for men) kilocalories in a day.

Now we can get back to weight. When you eat a meal, the food gets digested and is used by the body to grow, repair itself, and to provide the energy for your daily activities. This energy comes mainly from the fats and sugars in your food. If the energy in the food you eat is more than your body needs, then the extra is stored, mainly as fat, and you put on weight. If the energy in the food you eat is less than the body needs, then the body will use some of its stored fat to provide the extra energy needed and you lose weight. This is how calorie-controlled diets work. Your daily energy needs are worked out, and your daily food and drink contains LESS calories than you need. The body makes up the shortfall from its store of fat, and you lose weight.

Foods have been labelled with their calorie contents for many years. When it says that a chocolate biscuit contains 100 kilocalories, this means that when the biscuit is digested, your body can get 100 kilocalories of energy from it. That's enough to go for a 30 minute walk (see table page12). Put another way, it may take 30 seconds to eat the biscuit, but it takes a 30 minute walk to use up the kilocalories. If you eat the biscuit but don't take the walk, you'll put on about half an ounce in weight. That might not sound much, but one such biscuit a day for a month means that you'll put on a pound.

It should be clear that if you take in more calories than your body needs, you will put on weight, and if you take in fewer calories than your body needs, you will lose weight.

There are therefore 2 main ways to lose weight.

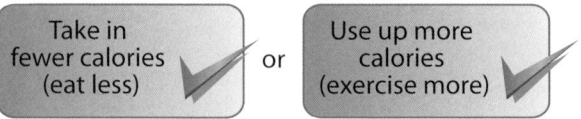

or, of course, do both.

It's not the purpose of this book to give advice on diet or on exercise programmes, since these things should be discussed with your health care team. Hopefully though, a better understanding of what calories are, and how they relate to weight, will make losing it easier.

It's also worth mentioning that regular exercise is really important for heart health but it's not a very efficient way of losing weight. A better way is to take in fewer calories.

You may ask – why should I bother? I know I'm overweight but I enjoy my food and I don't like exercise, and I feel OK, so what's the problem? The problem is that you are putting an extra strain on your body, especially your heart and blood vessels. You may well be able to continue with your lifestyle for many years, but the chances are that eventually your body will become unable to cope. Your heart may fail after years of extra work, your blood vessels may become blocked up, and you may develop diabetes, have a stroke or a heart attack.

There are lots of 'mays' here; these things may happen or they may not. What is certain however, is that overweight people have a far greater risk of becoming seriously ill than those who are not overweight. So it all comes down to how much you value your future health and whether you're prepared to act in such a way as to give yourself the best chance of a long and healthy life.

Coming back to the examples given in the Preface, would you stand next to someone on a crowded train who is coughing and sneezing; would you cross a busy road without looking out for traffic? If you would, then you may get away without catching a cold or being run over, but would you take the chance? Most people wouldn't.

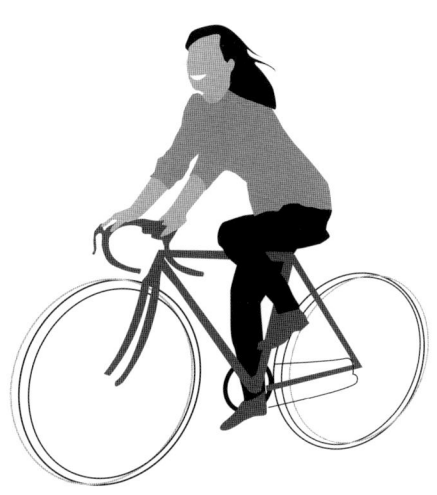

The Bottom Line

DON'T buy an exercise machine because after a while you'll stop using it. Ebay is full of such machines that are no longer used after an initial period of enthusiasm.

Unless you've got the determination to keep it going for the long term, DON'T join a gym or health club because after a while many people stop going and you'll have wasted most of your membership fee.

DON'T go on a diet because eventually you'll come off it and go back to your old eating habits and all the weight will come back.

DO try and cut down permanently on foods that you know are high in fat and sugar.

DO learn about healthy eating, and DO discuss this with your health care team.

And finally, DO buy an MP3 player, load it up with your CD collection, and go for a brisk walk at least every other day, and don't go back home until you've listened to 10 tracks. In other words, get used to doing some regular exercise, especially exercise that increases your heart rate.

2 Blood pressure

If you place your hand over your kitchen tap and turn on the hot water, you'll be able to stop the water from coming out if you push hard enough against the tap. Now try it with the cold water – you can't do it. Why not? The hot water is stored in a tank and the force (pressure) of the water as it comes out of the tap due to gravity is low enough for you to overcome it with your hand and so stop the water flow. The cold water however is pumped from the mains supply and is under far greater pressure – so great in fact that you can't stop it with your hand however hard you push.

What we've learnt here is that fluids are made to flow through a pipe by applying pressure at one end, either by gravity or by a pump. This is what happens in the body. The heart beats and pumps the blood round the body. As the heart beats, it forces an amount of blood into the circulation. The heart then relaxes before the next beat. It's obvious then that there is a higher pressure on the blood when the heart beats than when it has relaxed. These two pressures are the blood pressure. The first (higher) one is called the systolic pressure and the second (lower) one is called the diastolic pressure. When your blood pressure is measured, the results are given in the form 140/80; the first figure is the systolic pressure, and the second figure is the diastolic pressure.

How is blood pressure measured?

Blood pressure used to be measured by a mechanical device in which the pressure readings were shown on a glass tube filled with mercury but nowadays almost all doctors and nurses use the more convenient digital machines that give the readings on a display. You can even buy them at pharmacies for home measurement.

Blood pressure machines have an inflatable cuff that is placed round the upper arm (wrist cuffs are also available but are not as accurate), which is then inflated by the machine. This results in an increasing pressure being applied to the blood vessels in the arm, and eventually the pressure is high enough to stop the flow of blood (like the hot water in the tap).

The machine senses this and gradually releases the pressure until the blood flow starts again. These two points – the stopping and re-starting of the blood flow – represent the two blood pressure readings, and these are displayed on the digital screen.

What is a normal blood pressure?

This is an interesting question. By making measurements of blood pressure on many thousands of people from around the World, it has been possible to arrive at figures which can be considered as being 'normal'. The current medical guidelines for the UK, from the British Hypertension Society, are summarised in check list 3.

Check list 3 — Blood Pressure

Diagnosis	Blood pressure
Ideal	120/80 or less
Normal	130/85
High normal	130-139/85-89
Mildly high	140-159/90-99
Moderately high	160-179/100-109
Severely high	over 180/110

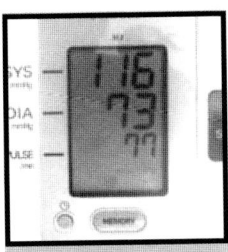

Healthy blood pressure readings (and pulse) in ideal range

If you have any form of heart disease, or you have diabetes, or you have a family history of these conditions, then your target ideal and normal figures should be lower than indicated in the check list. Your health care team will advise you. The basic rule is the lower the better (within reason of course; a very low blood pressure will make you faint).

It's important to realize that blood pressure varies a lot. If you take someone's blood pressure continually (they would be wearing a device that takes readings automatically every 30 minutes or so), you will see that it goes up and down during the day depending on what they are doing, and then usually goes down further at night. It can go up if you are nervous or anxious, so that while you are waiting for your doctor or nurse to take it, it goes up! By normal blood pressure, we mean the figures that would be obtained during ordinary daily activity and in a relaxed manner.

So, did you pass? If so, then well done. If not, don't worry because there are many things that can be done to get your blood pressure down to the recommended levels. First though, let's consider why blood pressure is so important.

Why is blood pressure important?

As we get older, our blood vessels start to become partially blocked with fatty deposits. This means that the same amount of blood has to be pushed through a narrower tube. To achieve this, it has to have a higher pressure. If you partially block the kitchen tap with your finger, the water comes out faster (higher pressure). If a blood vessel is half-blocked with fatty deposits, the pressure of the blood passing through the half-blocked vessel goes up 16 times!!

So why is high blood pressure important? There are lots of reasons: the heart has to work harder and is put under more strain, the blood vessels themselves can become damaged, and there is an increased risk of stroke, dementia, kidney damage, Peripheral Artery Disease (PAD) (page 41), and eye damage.

How do I know if I have high blood pressure?

You probably don't. High blood pressure usually occurs without any symptoms and it's possible for it to be present for many years and remain unnoticed. Sometimes, the effects of high blood pressure are first noticed during an eye examination where the optician sees changes in the small blood vessels in the back of the eye. It is therefore a very good idea for every adult to have their blood pressure checked at least once a year, or buy your own machine and measure your blood pressure at home. Most large pharmacies sell them. Buy one with an arm cuff rather than a wrist cuff since they are more reliable although they may be a bit more expensive. Ask the pharmacist for a model which has been approved by the British Hypertension Society.

Risk factors

Risk factors are things that make it more likely that something will happen. For example, smoking is a risk factor for lung cancer, because if you smoke your chances of getting lung cancer are increased. Not looking where you are going is a risk factor for bumping into something.

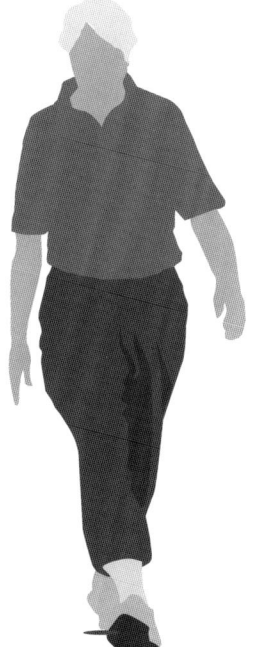

Some people are more at risk than others, and some lifestyle habits increase the risk. You can't do anything about your genetics, but you should at least be aware of them. A family history of heart disease and high blood pressure will mean an increased risk for you. Diabetes, smoking, obesity, high cholesterol, lack of exercise, and an unhealthy diet, are all risk factors for high blood pressure.

Salt is an easily avoidable risk factor. It has been known for years that salt increases blood pressure and that if you reduce the amount of salt in your food, then your blood pressure will fall. It is recommended that we eat no more than 6g (about one fifth of an ounce – a teaspoonful) of salt a day. This includes hidden salt in ready made foods as well as any salt that is added during cooking or at the table. Bear in mind also that if a food label gives the sodium content rather than the salt content, then this must be multiplied by 2.5 to give the weight of the salt. Salt is sodium chloride, and just giving the weight of the sodium is a sly move by the manufacturers to give the impression of a lower salt content than there really is.

Some sensible recommendations are:

- Buy unsalted or low-sodium versions of foods
- Restrict the eating of processed foods
- Don't cook with salt and don't add salt to food at the table – use herbs and spices instead

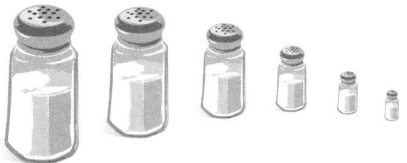

Treatment of high blood pressure

There are basically two types of treatment – lifestyle treatments and medical treatments. However, before treatment of any kind is begun, your health care team will need to make sure that you do really have high blood pressure. This will be done by taking measurements on 2 or 3 separate occasions. A diagnosis would never be made on the basis of just one reading.

Lifestyle treatments are things like giving up smoking, taking more exercise, losing weight, improving the diet, and avoiding salt and alcohol. These measures can all help to bring your blood pressure down but if it's not down far enough, then there is a large choice of medical treatments. Your doctor will discuss with you which drug or drugs are best suited to your particular situation.

Summary

Everyone has blood pressure since this is what makes the blood go around the body. As we get older, or as we settle into unhealthy lifestyles, our blood pressure can go up. If it gets above guideline figures shown in the check list, then it needs to be brought down, first by trying lifestyle treatments and then by medication. It's worth keeping a regular check on your blood pressure – high blood pressure has been called the silent killer because usually there are no symptoms

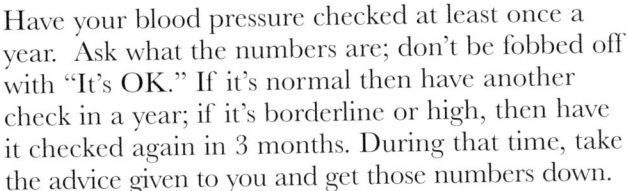

The Bottom Line

Have your blood pressure checked at least once a year. Ask what the numbers are; don't be fobbed off with "It's OK." If it's normal then have another check in a year; if it's borderline or high, then have it checked again in 3 months. During that time, take the advice given to you and get those numbers down.

3 Cholesterol

It's hard to avoid reading about cholesterol these days. It's mentioned regularly in the papers, and appears on most food labels. But what exactly is cholesterol?

Cholesterol is a fatty substance that is found in all animals. It is also present in small amounts in some plants. Although it regularly gets a bad press, cholesterol is actually very important to our good health. We all need it since it is used by the body to make certain hormones and to keep our cells in good condition. We couldn't live without cholesterol. It may surprise some people to learn that cholesterol is an important substance that is essential to life. However, back in 1957, it was discovered that people with too much cholesterol in their blood had an increased risk of getting heart disease.

Yes, we all need some cholesterol but as with many things, too much of a good thing can be bad. As an example, we might consider starting an old car on a cold morning. You pump the accelerator to get the petrol flowing so that the engine can fire. But you only need a certain amount; if you pump too much you will flood the engine and it won't start at all. Likewise, the body needs a certain amount of cholesterol so that it can produce the hormones we need and keep our cells in good condition. However, if there is too much, the extra builds up in the blood vessels causing clots, and you risk having a heart attack or stroke.

Where does the cholesterol in your blood come from? Some obviously comes from the food that you eat, and the food labels on the packaging will give you some information about this, but most of it (about three quarters) is made by your own liver.

Cholesterol levels

The importance of keeping your cholesterol levels under control has been known for over 50 years. Remember, everyone needs to have some cholesterol in their body, so

Before we go on to this however, one more thing needs to be explained. Being fatty, cholesterol cannot dissolve in the blood, so it is carried around the bloodstream in combination with other substances. We can simplify what is in reality quite a complicated process by saying that there are two main types of cholesterol moving around in the blood (see table below).

Good and bad cholesterol

Common name	Medical name
Good cholesterol	HDL cholesterol
Bad cholesterol	LDL cholesterol

See the Glossary for an explanation of what HDL and LDL mean.

It follows from this that what we should aim for is a high level of the GOOD cholesterol and a low level of the BAD cholesterol.

When you have your cholesterol measured (after an overnight fast), the results will usually contain 3 sets of numbers. These are the GOOD cholesterol (HDL), the BAD cholesterol (LDL), and the TOTAL cholesterol (confusingly, the total is not just the sum of the good and the bad!)

So we're now ready for our fourth check list.

Check list 4	Cholesterol		
Cholesterol Type	Desirable	Borderline	Too high or low
Total	less than 5.0	5.0 to 6.5	more than 6.5
Good (HDL)	more than 1.3	1.0 to 1.3	less than 1.0
Bad (LDL)	less than 2.6	2.6 to 4.2	more than 4.2

These figures are those that are used at the moment for normal healthy people. If you have diabetes, or have had a heart attack or stroke, or have a family history of heart problems, then your recommended levels will be different, your health care team will discuss this with you.

Your test results

If your results are not in the 'desirable' range, then you may be at an increased risk of a heart attack or stroke, and your doctor will recommend a course of action. If the figures are borderline only a little outside the desirable range, then the initial recommendation will probably be dietary and lifestyle. You know the deal – avoid fatty foods, take more exercise, and come back for another test in a few months.

If the results are in the 'too high or too low' range, or if diet and exercise haven't helped enough, then you will probably be prescribed a drug called a STATIN. These were discovered in the 1970s, and were first used as cholesterol-lowering drugs in 1987. They work by interfering with the mechanism by which the liver produces cholesterol. Think of statins as a tap – if there's too much water coming out of your shower head, then you'll turn the tap a bit to slow the water flow. Statins can be thought of as slowing down the production of cholesterol in the liver so less gets into the blood.

Many thousands of patients have been studied for many years, and for the vast majority statins are a safe and effective way to bring down high cholesterol levels and, most importantly, result in a reduced risk of death due to heart attacks and strokes. If there is a family history of heart disease, high blood pressure, stroke, or diabetes, or if you suffer from any of these conditions yourself, then it is even more important that cholesterol levels are reduced.

There are other fatty substances in the blood apart from cholesterol, and although these are also important as far as heart disease and good health are concerned, this book will just deal with cholesterol. If you want to learn more about fats in the blood, usually called LIPIDS, then it isn't hard to find information in books or on the internet, or by talking to your health care team.

The Bottom Line

High total cholesterol, high bad cholesterol, and low good cholesterol, are all associated with an increased risk of heart disease and stroke. Get yours checked, and ask for your numbers. Get them back to the recommended values and keep them there.

4 Stroke

Stroke is the third commonest cause of death in the United Kingdom, and there are about 130,000 cases every year. About a third of patients either die or need constant care.

A stroke is caused by a sudden interruption to the blood flow in the brain. This can be caused by two things – a clot (which blocks the blood flow) or a bleed from a burst blood vessel (which means the blood doesn't go where it should and does go where it shouldn't). Either way, parts of the brain are suddenly starved of blood and oxygen.

The medical name for a stroke caused by a blood clot is an ischaemic stroke, and that for a stroke caused by a bleed is a haemorrhagic stroke. Strokes caused by clots are by far the commonest and account for more than 80% of all strokes.

We should mention here another type of stroke, called a Transient Ischaemic Attack (TIA), which is a sort of mini-stroke. It's caused by a temporary blockage in one of the arteries in the brain, but the blockage disappears quite quickly as do the effects on the patient. We'll come back to TIAs shortly, since they do have an importance.

The effects of a stroke are very variable, since it depends which part of the brain has been affected. These could include weakness on one side of the body, disturbed balance and/or vision, and difficulty with speech, swallowing, memory, or emotions.

Many patients make a full or partial recovery but sadly some will remain disabled in some way, or may even die.

Because the effects are so varied, the best way to diagnose a stroke is by a brain scan.

Risk factors

There are some things that do give us an increased risk of having a stroke but which we can do nothing about. These include our age, sex, ethnicity, and family history. However, the good news is that there are still plenty of things that we can do to minimize our chances of having a stroke.

High blood pressure is the number 1 risk factor for stroke. If you have high (above 130/85) blood pressure, then your risk for stroke is increased 7 times. Not controlling high blood pressure is a major cause of strokes.

Smoking increases your chances of having a stroke 4 times.

Abnormal heart rhythms especially atrial fibrillation, can cause blood clots to form. These can cause a stroke if they reach the brain (Atrial fibrillation, AF, is the commonest of various conditions in which there is an irregular heartbeat. In AF, the top chambers of the heart, called the atria, beat faster than the bottom ones, resulting in an irregular blood flow and feelings of weakness and tiredness. Treatment is usually by drugs or minor surgical procedures).

Weight control and exercise are very important. As stated previously, if you're overweight your blood pressure rises and this will increase the risk of having a burst blood vessel (haemorrhagic stroke).

Oral contraceptives on their own are not a serious risk factor, but this does become important if you are also a smoker or you have high blood pressure. Therefore, if you are on the Pill, it is important that you take especial care to keep your blood pressure under control, and not to smoke.

Transient Ischaemic Attacks (TIAs) often called Mini-strokes, are a warning sign for a possible future stroke. Nearly 10% of patients who have a TIA will have a full stroke within a year. Any sudden and temporary loss of vision in one eye, double vision, difficulty in speaking or swallowing, or numbness or weakness to one side of the body, should be investigated immediately. Don't be fooled into thinking that the effects are unimportant because they only lasted for a few minutes or even seconds. You need an urgent brain and possibly a carotid (neck) artery scan, and many hospitals now have a special neurology service for people who have had a TIA. It's been said that TIA could also stand for Take Immediate Action.

If you think that this is over the top and unnecessary, then consider the following. You're driving along and approaching a traffic jam. You apply the brakes but nothing happens – the pedal goes right down to the floor and the car keeps on going. You keep pressing the pedal when suddenly the brakes work again and you slow down. The whole episode only lasted a few seconds.

What would you do?

 1 Nothing, as the problem has corrected itself.

Wrong

Brakes don't mend themselves and it may happen again and stay broken. There's obviously a fault with the braking system that needs immediate attention.

 2 Nothing, but if it happens again then have it checked.

Wrong

As in 1, the next time it happens it may stay broken, and you may be driving down a hill or approaching a Zebra crossing. Or the edge of a cliff.

 3 Have it checked immediately.

Right

Head injury

Although not directly related to a stroke, it's worth mentioning here that any head injury, perhaps due to a fall, motor or industrial accident, should receive urgent medical attention even if the casualty insists otherwise. This is especially the case if there has been a loss of consciousness. A bleed in the brain needs immediate specialist treatment, and can only be reliably diagnosed with a brain scan. Any unnecessary delay could have tragic consequences, as in the sad case of the actress Natasha Richardson who refused hospital treatment after a skiing accident in which she had hit her head, and died soon afterwards.

This is because there is a relatively short period of time (hours) before any damage to the brain becomes irreversible.

Treatment

The most important thing is for someone, and this could be you, to realize that you may have had a stroke, and to get you to a hospital equipped with a stroke unit as soon as possible. A scan will determine the type of stroke, and if it turns out to be due to a blockage, then clot-busting drugs must be given within a few hours of the stroke. Later than that, and they may have no effect since damage to the brain will already have been done. Surgery can also be an option in some cases.

Haemorrhagic (bleeding) strokes are generally treated with blood pressure lowering and sometimes, surgery. Rehabilitation forms an important part of treatment after a stroke.

The Stroke Association have recently (2009) launched their FAST campaign to help in recognizing if someone has had a stroke. It requires an assessment of 3 symptoms:

FACE
has their eye or mouth drooped; can they smile?

ARM
can they raise both arms?

SPEECH
can they speak clearly and understand you?

TIME
if any of these tests are failed, it's time to call 999.

The Bottom Line

Look after your general health, especially your weight, blood pressure, cholesterol levels, and blood sugar. Take regular exercise. If you think that you or someone with you may have had a stroke or a TIA, get them to the nearest stroke unit as soon as possible.

5 Diabetes

Diabetes is a common condition and is becoming more so. Worldwide, it is estimated that there are close to 200 million people with diabetes; in the UK over 2 million people have diabetes and a further half a million or so have it but don't know it – yet. Probably due to genetic reasons, South Asian and black African Caribbean people have a 4 or 5 times greater risk of developing Type 2 diabetes compared to Europeans. Up to 25% of South Asian adults over the age of 50 have diabetes. So, what is diabetes?

The body needs a source of energy in order to carry out all of its functions and this source of energy is glucose (usually referred to in lay terms as sugar). Glucose is obtained from the food that we eat, especially the carbohydrates such as bread, rice and potatoes, and ends up in the bloodstream. From there, it can be absorbed into the cells and tissues that need it, such as the brain, liver, heart, muscles etc.

In a normal healthy person, the amount of glucose in the blood is controlled to between about 4 and 6 units. This control is due to the presence of a substance called insulin. Insulin is made by the body in the pancreas. Diabetes is a condition in which either there isn't enough insulin in the body or it doesn't do its job properly. This results in high levels of glucose in the blood (more than 7 units), and in too little glucose reaching the cells that need it for energy.

There are two types of diabetes, known as Type 1 and Type 2 diabetes.

Type 1 diabetes usually develops in thin young children although it can also occur in adults. It is caused by a partial or complete lack of insulin. About 10% of people with diabetes have the Type 1 variety.

Type 2 diabetes usually develops in overweight adults over the age of 40, but can also occur in adolescents and even in children. It is a particular problem in South Asian and African Caribbean people, who can develop it in their teens. It occurs when the pancreas either doesn't make enough insulin, or when the insulin doesn't work properly. This is called insulin resistance. About 90% of people with diabetes have Type 2.

The end result is therefore the same in both types of diabetes: the cells that need it cannot use glucose for the production of energy, and the level of glucose builds up in the blood, sometimes to very high, and possibly dangerous levels.

Symptoms and diagnosis

Common symptoms of diabetes include thirst, excessive urination, frequent skin infections including thrush, tiredness and weight loss. Less commonly there is pins and needles in the legs and feet, and blurring of vision. The diagnosis is made after a blood test which measures the amount of glucose in your blood after an overnight fast.

So now we reach our fifth check list.

Check list 5	Diabetes		
	Normal	Borderline	Diabetes
fasting blood glucose	6.1 or less	6.1 to 6.9	7.0 or more

If your blood glucose measurement is 6.1 or less, then that is normal and you do not have diabetes. It's worth remembering however that most people who don't have diabetes have fasting glucose levels of between about 4 to 5. If it is in the borderline range of 6.1 to 6.9, then you have what is called impaired fasting glucose. This isn't diabetes but it isn't quite normal either, and it may develop into diabetes later.

You may need a Glucose Tolerance Test (you are given a glucose drink and blood tests are taken every 30 minutes to see how your body copes with the glucose in the drink). This will enable your health care team to decide whether you need any further tests or treatment.

If your fasting blood glucose is 7.0 or more, then the test should be repeated to make sure about the result. If it is still 7.0 or more, then you do have diabetes, and your health care team will talk to you about treatments.

Treatments

For anyone with diabetes, it is essential that they follow the lifestyle and dietary advice given by their health care team.

If you have Type 1 diabetes, then you will need insulin injections for life. With modern injection pens and other devices, this isn't nearly as bad as you might think, but it does require commitment and family support.

Patients with Type 2 diabetes can often control their blood glucose levels by following dietary and lifestyle advice, and may need no medication at all. Should this not be sufficient, then there is a wide selection of drugs available, most of them in tablet form, though some patients will require injections.

The single most important thing is that your blood glucose levels remain in the normal range.

Complications

Complications can be thought of as unwanted side effects, and are usually divided into two types. Doctors use the term acute to describe symptoms that occur quickly over a short time scale, and the term chronic for those symptoms that appear more slowly but last for much longer.

The acute complications of diabetes usually result from either too little or too much glucose in the blood. Too little (hypoglycaemia) is usually caused by missed or delayed food, too much medication or insulin, or too much physical activity. It can result in confusion, aggressive behaviour, sweating, fits and rarely coma. Treatment is easy and involves no more than a sugary drink or snack to bring the glucose levels up again. Too much glucose in the blood (hyperglycaemia) is usually caused by too little medication, or another illness or infection. This may not be a problem over the short term, but if blood glucose levels remain high for longer, several hours say, this can lead to a hospital admission.

The chronic complications of diabetes can occur over months or even years. They include problems in the eyes, the kidney (chronic kidney disease – see below), and the nerves to the legs and feet. Heart attacks are the commonest complication of Type 2 diabetes. The best way of preventing these chronic complications is to ensure that the blood glucose, blood cholesterol, and blood pressure levels stay within the ranges specified by your health care team. This involves taking your medication as and when directed, keeping your weight under control, and taking regular exercise.

Peripheral Arterial Disease (PAD)
(also called Peripheral Vascular Disease, PVD)

Peripheral Arterial Disease (PAD) is caused by a narrowing of the blood vessels in the legs (it can also occur in the arms but this is very unusual). It becomes more common in older people as their blood vessels become partially blocked with fatty deposits.

People with diabetes are especially at risk of PAD, but other risk factors include the usual suspects of obesity, lack of exercise, smoking, high blood pressure and cholesterol levels, and a family history of heart disease.

A major symptom of PAD is pain in the legs on walking, known as claudication. It's caused by the leg muscles becoming partially starved of oxygen due to the narrowed artery.

In very severe cases where the blood supply is greatly reduced, there may be leg pain even at rest. If left untreated, the blood supply to the foot may become so reduced that the tissue actually dies and the foot becomes gangrenous and may need to be amputated.

It's obvious therefore that any leg pain during or after mild exercise should be reported to your health care team, especially if you have any of the risk factors mentioned above.

Chronic Kidney Disease (CKD)

This can also be a complication of diabetes. The kidneys are responsible for removing waste products from the blood, and so are essential to health. In chronic kidney disease, the kidneys gradually become less able to do their job properly, and the end result can be end stage kidney failure. To prevent waste products building up in the blood, which would quickly be fatal, the patient will need lifelong dialysis, or a kidney transplant.

Summary

There are definite lifestyle risk factors that can increase your chances of getting diabetes. These include being overweight, taking insufficient exercise, and eating or drinking lots of sugary foods and drinks. Make sure that your lifestyle doesn't put you at risk.

The Bottom Line

Keep your weight under control, take regular exercise, don't eat or drink too many sugary foods or drinks, and don't smoke. Don't ignore possible symptoms of diabetes - if you regularly have the urge to urinate, if you feel excessively thirsty, if you feel tired, and if you sweat a lot, then have a blood test to see if your glucose levels are normal. If it turns out that you have diabetes, make sure that you follow the advice given to you. Above all, keep your blood sugar and blood pressure levels under control to help reduce the chances of complications. In a nutshell, watch your numbers.

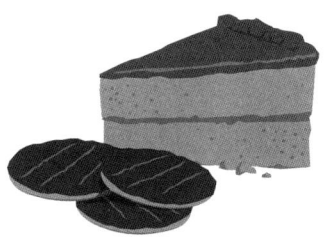

6 Cancer

The mere mention of the word cancer fills most people with dread since they assume it is a death sentence. It's certainly true that some cancers, such as those of the lung, breast, and colon, are significant causes of death but new treatments and early detection have resulted in real improvements. For patients, this means longer survival and sometimes a complete cure.

So what exactly is cancer? All livings things are made of cells. This is a photograph of some human skin cells.

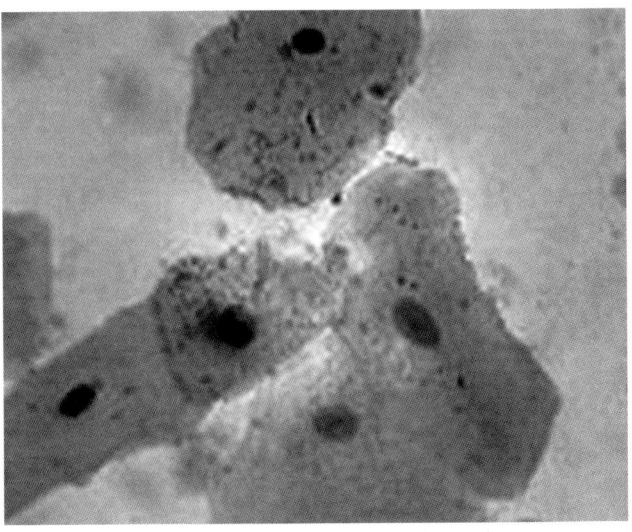

Cells are very small, so small that they can only be seen under a microscope. Some living things, such as bacteria, are made up of just one cell, whereas large animals and humans have many billions of cells. Each part of the body has its own type of cell, so that a liver cell, for example, is different in shape and size from a skin cell. Obviously, they also have different functions.

Living things grow and repair themselves when their cells divide into two, and then into 4 etc. This process is controlled so that the cells only divide when necessary. Normally, cells stay in their own place. For example, liver cells are only ever found in the liver.

Sometimes this control can go wrong, and the cells start to divide more than they should. A lump of cells is formed, and this is a cancer. If the lump (cancer) stays in its place, for example, the liver, then it is benign. This means that it is a local problem only, and the lump can usually be treated with drugs or by surgery. If however the cells in the lump start to spread out of the liver to other parts of the body, then it is called malignant, and this can be serious. Treatment with drugs or by surgery is still possible but the earlier this is done the better.

Think of a lump of cancer cells as a walled city. If the cells stay within the walls, then it is easier to treat the problem and be cured. If the cells get out of the walled city and spread around the neighbouring regions (the rest of the body), then it becomes much harder to treat the problem. Clearly, it is better to begin the treatment as soon as possible, before too many cells have gained a foothold outside the walls.

Cancer has many causes. These include such things as family history which obviously we can do nothing about, and our lifestyle, such as smoking, which we certainly can do something about. There are more than 200 different types of cancer but about half of all new cases consist of just 4 types – breast, lung, colon, and prostate. Here is a chart showing the 20 commonest cancers in the UK.

There were about 366,000 new cases of cancer diagnosed in the UK in 2005, and 156,000 of them, nearly half, were made up of breast, lung, colon, and prostate.

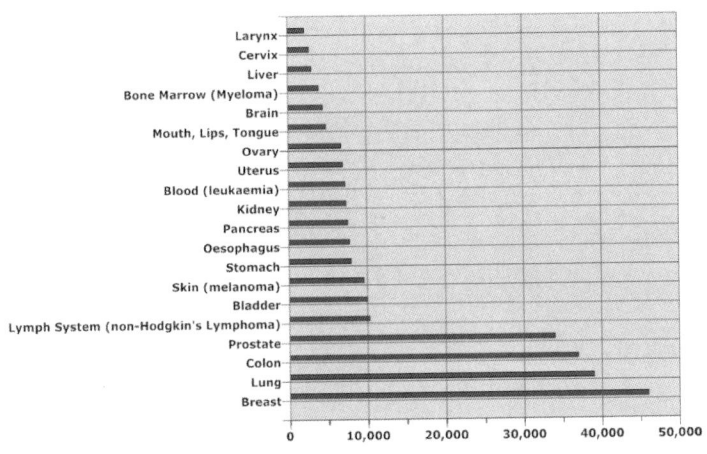

The 20 most common cancers diagnosed in the UK in 2005. The figures are the number of cases and are taken from Cancer UK data.

Here are some things that we can do to reduce our risks of getting cancer.

1 Try and prevent it in the first place

How? Many cancers have a known cause.

Most cases of lung cancer are caused by smoking cigarettes. Those who don't believe this are fooling themselves. The link between lung cancer and smoking has been known for over 50 years. So the answer here is DON'T SMOKE. If you do, then STOP. If you find this difficult, get help from your health care team.

Cancer of the large intestine, colon cancer, has a genetic component about which nothing can be done but there are other causes which can be avoided. Most of these are dietary in origin. You should avoid fatty foods and chemically preserved and smoked meats, and should eat plenty of fibre-rich foods, and fruits and vegetables.

If there is any trace of blood in your stools then an urgent medical appointment is essential. It may mean nothing, or it may be an early indication of something serious.

Don't ignore this possible warning sign. If you live in an area where your Health Authority offers a colon cancer screening service, then take up this valuable offer. The test is done by you in your own home, and just involves sending a small sample of your stools, in a special pack which is provided, to a laboratory.

Malignant melanoma, a form of skin cancer, is on the increase, with about 9,000 new cases in the UK each year and about 2,000 deaths. Almost all are related to too much exposure to the Sun. So it makes sense to limit your exposure especially if you are fair-skinned and in a hot climate. Use sun protection lotions. Remember though that these won't prevent sun burn; they just delay it. Be especially careful with children.

Sun beds also emit rays which penetrate deeply into the skin. Don't use them. They are probably as dangerous as cigarettes and many specialists think that they should be banned or at least subject to greater controls. If you want to have a tanned appearance, there are now plenty of harmless tanning creams that will give you a very lifelike tan.

If you notice any change in the appearance of a mole on your skin, get it checked out immediately.

Breast cancer is diagnosed in over 40,000 women (and a few hundred men) in the UK every year. As part of the National Breast Cancer Screening programme, every woman between the ages of 50 and 70 is entitled to a mammogram examination every 3 years.

A mammogram is a painless procedure in which each breast is X rayed to see if there are any abnormalities that need to be investigated further. If you are invited to have a mammogram, you should take this up. If there is a problem, then you want to know about as soon as possible.

In reality, many breast problems are first noticed by the women themselves. There are several reasons for this. You may be too young or too old to be in the screening programme or the symptoms may become apparent during the 3 year interval between mammograms.

It is very important for women to undertake regular self-examination of their breasts. The NHS has a 5 point breast awareness code:

know what is normal for you
look at your breasts and feel your breasts
know what changes to look for (size, shape, feel)
report any changes immediately
attend the breast screening clinic if you are eligible

If there are any worrying signs then your health care team should be contacted immediately. In the vast majority of cases there will be nothing to worry about but if there is, it needs to be dealt with as soon as possible.

Cervical cancer affects about 3,000 women every year and around half of them will eventually die from the disease. Cervical cancer is primarily caused by infection with a virus which is usually transmitted by sexual contact. The more sexual partners a women has, the more likely it is that she will encounter someone who is infected with the virus.

From the age of 20 in Scotland, Wales and Northern Ireland, and 25 in England, women who have ever been sexually active should have regular cervical smears. This is just a simple screening test to look for any early changes in the cells that may lead to cancer years later. If any abnormal cells are found, they can be removed and the chances of cancer developing are then reduced. Vaccines are now available which protect against the commonest viruses (HPV 16 and HPV 18) which together cause about 70% of all cervical cancers. Much like vaccination against polio and measles has practically wiped out these diseases, the new vaccines are likely to prevent significant numbers of cases of cervical cancer.

The publicity surrounding the death from cervical cancer of 27 year old Jade Goody in March 2009 led to an increase in awareness of this disease, and a recognition of the importance of cervical screening.

Prostate cancer is the commonest male cancer in the UK and accounts for about a quarter of all male cancers. Over 30,000 men are diagnosed with prostate cancer each year, and there are about 10,000 deaths annually. It is more common in older men (over the age of 70) and is rare under the age of 50 although some ethnic groups, for example, Africans and African Caribbeans can develop it at an earlier age. As with several other cancers, a family history will increase an individual's personal risk.

The classical symptoms include the need to urinate frequently, especially at night, difficulty or pain while urinating, a decreased flow of urine, and sometimes a feeling that there is still more urine to come.

However, just having some or all of these symptoms doesn't mean that you have prostate cancer; there are other non-cancerous conditions that can cause similar symptoms, one of which is a benign (non-malignant) increased prostate size.

If any of these symptoms are present, you must have an immediate medical examination to find out the cause of the problem. The doctor will probably want to examine the size of your prostate gland (this is called a digital rectal examination – it may not be very elegant but it doesn't hurt and only lasts a few seconds). This may be followed by a blood test. If this is positive, it may indicate a cancer but this can only be confirmed after a small operation (biopsy).

Prostate cancers are generally slow-growing, so early detection and treatment often results in cures. The message therefore is: don't ignore worrying signs.

Testicular cancer is not that common and only 1 to 2 of every 100 cancers diagnosed in men are testicular cancers. It is mentioned here because there is a link between the development of testicular cancer and undescended testicles. Both testicles should be in position in the scrotum by the time a baby is 1 year old. If this is not the case, then advice and treatment should be sought. If this is delayed, there could be an increased risk of developing testicular cancer at a later stage.

2 Have a screening test if you are in a high risk group by virtue of age, job, ethnicity or family history.

Examples of basic screening tests are mammography (and self-examination) for breast lumps, blood tests for prostate cancer, smears for cervical caner, and blood in the stools for colon cancer.

3 Don't ignore worrying symptoms

Worrying symptoms would include the following: weight loss for no apparent reason, lumps (such as in the breast or the testicles), change in bowel habits, change in appearance of skin moles from smooth to jagged edges, blood in the stools or urine, coughing up blood, etc. Don't take the old-fashioned attitude that if there's something wrong then you don't want to know. The chances are that it's nothing serious, but if it is then the sooner treatment begins, the higher the chance that you'll be cured. Unlike most aches and pains, cancer doesn't get better on its own.

Smoking

Smoking is seriously bad for your health. It causes lung cancer and other lung diseases, makes you more prone to serious respiratory infections, and increases your risk of developing heart disease, strokes, and diabetes. If you're still not convinced, have a look at these two illustrations. One shows a normal healthy pair of lungs and the other shows a pair of lungs blackened and shrivelled by tobacco smoke and tar and advanced cancer, and a dead owner. You know which is which!

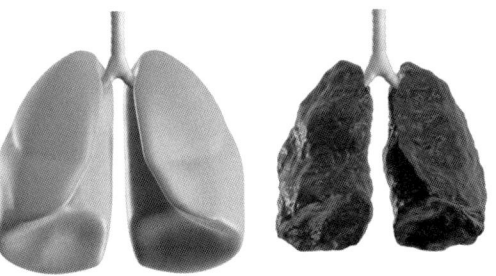

Illustrations showing normal and diseased lungs. Images © fotolia

If you're a smoker, here's a little experiment you can do yourself: inhale your cigarette through a piece of tissue and see how brown it gets after just one puff. That's what's going into your delicate lungs.

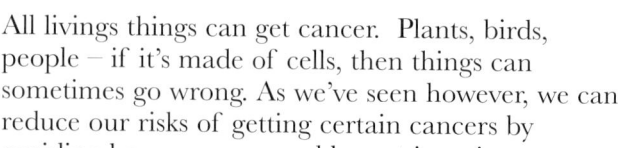

The Bottom Line

All livings things can get cancer. Plants, birds, people – if it's made of cells, then things can sometimes go wrong. As we've seen however, we can reduce our risks of getting certain cancers by avoiding known causes and by not ignoring any worrying signs.

Learn about lifestyle changes that can reduce the risk of getting cancer. Learn how to examine yourself for lumps and changes in mole appearance, and do it regularly. Have a screening test if you are in a high risk group. Get immediate medical advice if you develop any symptoms that worry you. Don't smoke. And remember this formula:

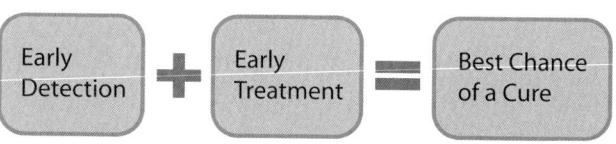

Early Detection + Early Treatment = Best Chance of a Cure

7 Will I have a heart attack?

Obviously, a question like this can't be answered with any degree of certainty, and, it has to be said, there are some people who may prefer not to know. However, for those that do have an interest in their likely future health, science and medicine can offer some guidelines.

On the basis of many years of research on many thousands of people, it's now possible to estimate your personal chances of having a heart attack or stroke within the next 10 years. Your own doctor can do this calculation for you, if you ask for it. He or she will need to have the results of recent blood and other tests, and can then look up the results on a chart or on a computer program.

You should realize that this is just a guide, based on your current health, and on things like your blood pressure, cholesterol, and on your past medical history. It's a bit like a garage telling you that your car will probably be needing new tyres within a year. That may indeed turn out to be true but, depending on how the car is used, the tyres may last for a bit longer than that. Or they may wear out after just 6 months. It's just a guide that in the not-too-distant future you will probably need new tyres.

So here's our sixth Check List.

Check list 6 | Heart Attack

Chart to estimate the risk of a fatal heart attack within the next 10 years

Reproduced from European Heart Journal. 2007:28,2375-2414 by kind permission of Oxford University Press

You will see that this chart consists of 4 columns each made up of 5 coloured squares for different ages. The two left hand columns are for women, and the two right hand ones are for men. Each set is then divided into separate columns for smokers and non-smokers. To use the chart, you must first select the correct column - man or woman; smoker or non-smoker. Then select the square that most closely matches your age.

The next stage involves knowing your blood pressure and your total cholesterol readings. The numbers up the left hand side are the systolic blood pressure (higher) numbers; for example if your blood pressure readings are 145/95 then it's the 145 you need. The numbers along the bottom are for your total cholesterol.

As an example, let's use the chart for a 58 year old male smoker, with a systolic blood pressure reading of 157 and a total cholesterol reading of 6.4. His square is in the fourth column from the left (men; smoker), second large square down (60; this is the nearest one to his age). You'll see that each large square is made up of 20 smaller coloured squares with numbers in them. The nearest blood pressure to his 157 on the scale is 160. This is the second row down within his large square. The nearest cholesterol reading to his 6.4 on the scale is 6. This is the third small square from the left. This has the number 17 in it. What this means is that he has a 17% risk of having a fatal heart attack within the next 10 years.

Had his blood pressure and his cholesterol been lower, say 138 and 5.3, then his risk would have been 10%. Quite a difference!

Finally, we need to try and put these risk percentages into context. Naturally, there will always be some risk of dying from a heart attack, but how typical is our sample patient with his 17% risk?

Look at the small charts below. Our patient is a smoker with a systolic blood pressure of 157 (nearest on scale is 160) and a total cholesterol of 6.4 (nearest on scale is 6). His small square is red and has a 6 in it. The lowest number in any square is a 1 (the green squares which are for non-smokers with low blood pressure and low to medium cholesterol). Our patient's number 6 means that his risk is 6 times higher than someone of his age who would be in a green square, that is, someone whose blood pressure and cholesterol levels are no worse than 'high normal'.

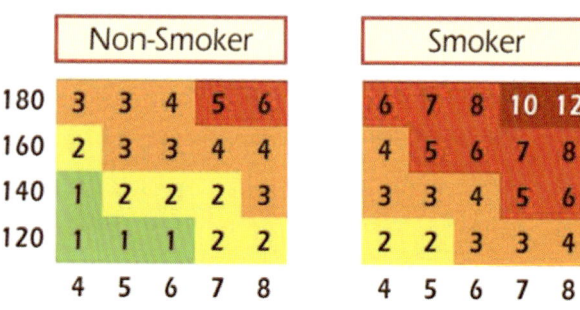

Chart to estimate the relative risk of a fatal heart attack within the next 10 years - compared to someone of the same age

Reproduced from European Heart Journal. 2007:28,2375-2414 by kind permission of Oxford University Press

All these charts are based on the medical histories of 250,000 European patients who were studied for several years. Your personal risk may be higher if you have any genetic risk factors (history of heart disease either personally or in your family, or if you are South Asian or black African Caribbean), or if your blood pressure and cholesterol numbers have been lowered by drugs.

There are quite a few such charts, each produced by different organisations in different countries. They vary in their detail but overall will give similar results. The ones in this book have been chosen because they are very clear and quite easy to use by non-medical people. But they are only a guide.

Similar charts for predicting the risk of a stroke are also available.

8 Eye tests

The basic eyesight test involves reading a series of letters of differing sizes, and noting the smallest size that can be read clearly and accurately. However, apart from making sure that your eyesight is at its best, with glasses if you need them, a professional eye examination also gives an early warning about various other conditions.

High blood pressure is often first noticed by your optician rather than your Health Care Team because there will be tell-tale signs in the small blood vessels in the eye. These would be examined during every routine eye test. If your optician does detect any changes that might suggest high blood pressure, see your Health Care Team or nurse. Remember, high blood pressure usually has no symptoms, so don't neglect the advice of your optician.

Diabetes can also sometimes be spotted first during an eye examination, again by your optician noticing changes in the back of the eye. As above, don't ignore your optician's advice. Glaucoma is caused by an increased pressure inside the eyeball which can damage the optic nerve. In its early stages there are no symptoms but if left untreated, can lead to blindness. If your optician does detect any changes that might suggest high blood pressure, then you should arrange to have this checked.

If you need it, treatment would consist of eye drops with possible surgery later if necessary. It's especially important to have this test done if you have a family history of glaucoma. It is more common in those over the age of 40 and in people who have diabetes.

There are several other rarer medical conditions that can also be picked up during an eye examination. It is important to realize therefore that an eye examination actually examines much more than just the eyes.

9 Lung function tests

Lung diseases (cancer, infections, COPD – chronic obstructive pulmonary disease, almost always due to smoking) are major killers, and it is worth having your lung function measured every now and then, especially if you are asthmatic or have any worries about your breathing. The simplest test is to measure your peak flow rate – this is your maximum ability to breathe out. The test can be carried out by your Health Care Team, or you can even buy a meter and do it at home.

The test is performed with a peak flow meter which is basically a tube that you blow in to, with an inner disk attached to a pointer. Markings on a scale show how far the disk has moved, and this is known as your peak flow rate. A value of between 400 and 600 (measured as litres per minute – L/min) would be considered normal. The values will however vary within this range according to your sex, age, height, and general fitness.

Medical advice should be sought if peak flow rate values are consistently below 400 L/min.

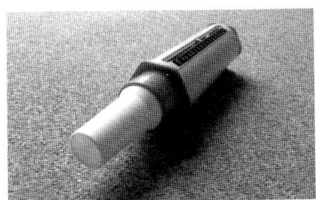

peak flow meter

10 Your own MOT

Medical and Optical Tests check list

So now that we've almost come to the end of the book, are you in good shape? Would you pass your MOT (Medical and Optical Tests)? Our final check list will allow you to put in your own test results and see at a glance which parts of your body haven't passed. Take the appropriate action, where possible, and get as many through the next test as possible. There's no official certificate if you pass all the tests but there is something much better – the knowledge that you have done all that you can to live a longer and healthier life.

This checklist has some sample results to demonstrate how it should be used. The column showing DESIRABLE values contains the range of numbers that would be obtained from normal healthy white adults.

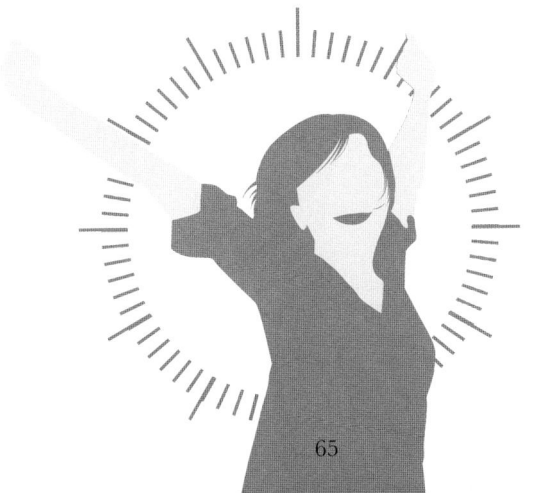

Check list 7: Your own MOT

System	Sample Result	Pass/Fail	Your Result	Desirable
Bodywork				
Waist circumference (female)	94cm	✗		88cm
Waist circumference (male)	98cm	✓		102cm
Engine				
Blood pressure	150/95	✗		140/85 or less
Total cholesterol	6.1	✗		5.2 or less
Good (HDL) cholesterol	0.9	✗		more than 1.3
Bad (LDL) cholesterol	3.7	✗		less than 2.6
10 year risk of heart attack	20%	✗		pass if normal for age
30 mins. of exercise 3 times a week	no	✗		
Lights				
Eye test in last 2 years	no	✗		
Fuel & cooling systems				
Excessive thirst	no	✓		
Excessive urination	no	✓		
Fasting blood sugar	4.7	✓		4 - 6
5 portions fruit and vegetables per day	yes	✓		
Less than 6g sodium chloride per day	yes	✓		
3 portions oily fish per week	no	✗		
Emissions				
Smoker	yes	✗		
Lung function (peak flow rate)	280	✗		400 - 600

11 Vitamins and supplements

We should say something about vitamins and food supplements because they are often in the news and advertised as being good for you. Is that really true?

It's been known for a long time that eating certain foods could prevent certain illnesses. For example, the Ancient Egyptians knew that night blindness could be cured by eating liver. In the 18th Century, it was found that eating citrus fruits like lemons and limes could prevent scurvy, a disease in which wounds do not heal properly, gums bleed, there is much pain, and eventually death. This resulted in Royal Navy sailors on long voyages being given limes, hence the nickname 'Limeys'. Later discoveries made it clear that some foods contained other factors apart from the well-known fats, carbohydrates and proteins, and that these 'other factors' were essential to good health. They were called 'vitamines'; nowadays the word is spelt without the 'e' – VITAMINS.

Vitamins are named with letters of the alphabet, and there are over a dozen that have been known for at least 60 years. All are needed for good health. However, we don't need much of them. As an example, the recommended daily requirement of vitamin A is just under 1 milligram (mg). That's about one thirty thousandth of an ounce. Put another way, one ounce would last one person for over 80 years!

Similar calculations apply to the other vitamins. So although we do need them to keep healthy, we don't need much. Why then is the vitamin and supplement market so buoyant? In the UK, it is worth around £400 million a year.

Vitamin and supplement manufacturers and suppliers are making a fortune selling their products to millions of people, the overwhelming majority of whom don't need them. The marketing is clever and includes some persuasive arguments, such as:

Modern methods of food production mean that there is less 'goodness' in our food so we need to take extra vitamins and supplements to compensate.

As we get older, our bodies need more vitamins and minerals so we need to take extra.

Optimum health is only achieved if we take more than the recommended daily allowance (RDA).

This last point is made by various vitamin and supplement companies. Their message is that although the RDA of vitamin A, for example, is 800 micrograms, you'd be healthier if you consume 3 times that amount, so you'd better buy our tablets. Is that true?

As was discussed at the beginning of this chapter, vitamins were discovered when it was noticed that some diseases could be cured by eating certain foods. Here is a brief list:

Disease	Vitamin Needed
Night Blindness (hard to see in dim light)	vitamin A
Beri-Beri (fatigue; nerve damage; death)	vitamin B1
Pellagra (stomach, skin, and nerve disorders; death)	vitamin B3
Scurvy (bleeding gums and internal organs; death)	vitamin C
Rickets (poor bone development)	vitamin D

These diseases are very rare in the UK and in industrialized countries unless there are significant dietary restrictions. For example, the increasing use of pre-packaged and 'fast' food, combined with little or no fresh fruit and little exposure to the sun, can all lead to people becoming vitamin deficient. If this describes your diet and lifestyle then you may benefit from extra vitamins. Talk to your health care team.

So what does this tell us? It tells us that most people get all the vitamins they need to stay healthy from their diet, provided of course that it is a balanced one including fruit and vegetables and a source of protein (meat or vegetarian alternatives). Food may well be less fresh nowadays, but as long as we eat enough of the right types, and also get a certain amount of sunshine on our skin (which is how the body produces vitamin D), we'll still get enough vitamins to prevent us from getting deficiency diseases like scurvy etc.

But what about the idea that the recommended amounts of vitamins are actually not enough for perfect health, and that more is better?

Despite what the health food manufacturers and suppliers would have you believe, the answer is the vast majority of cases is NO. There's just no evidence that, for most people, taking more than the recommended amounts of vitamins has any benefits at all. One exception is that pregnant women should take extra FOLIC ACID to ensure the health of their baby.

In most cases, not only will extra vitamins not do you any good, in some cases they can actually do you harm since they can cause liver and nerve damage if taken in excess. They'll also cost you a lot of money. Have a look at the Food Standards Agency website for some authoritative and unbiased advice (details in the Appendix).

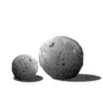
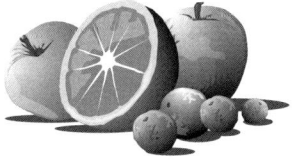

Think of a car engine with all its moving parts. The engine needs a supply of oil to lubricate these parts, and if the engine runs out of oil, it will begin to overheat and eventually stop. Keeping your oil topped up to the mark is therefore essential for the good health of your car engine, but overfilling it does no good at all. It is a waste of money and can even do harm by getting into places where it shouldn't be.

The body also needs a supply of minerals and various other substances to keep it going, and these come under the general heading of Supplements. Again we don't need much of them, and will get all that we do need from our food.

Finally, there is a whole collection of other substances which can be bought from health food shops or online, but for which there is little evidence that we need them. You could spend a lot of money on these products and get no benefits at all. One exception is oily fish, such as herring and mackerel, which are rich in substances known as omega 3 fatty acids, and it has been known for a long time that eating oily fish does offer health benefits, especially in relation to heart disease. It is recommended therefore, that a healthy diet should include 2 or 3 portions of oily fish per week. If you can't do that, then it is possible to buy capsules that contain these omega 3 fatty acids.

Cholesterol-lowering foodstuffs, such as Benecol® and Pro-Activ®, should also be mentioned. These contain plant extracts that can lower cholesterol a bit, and are usually supplied as spreads for bread or as yoghurts or drinks. They can lower cholesterol by about 10% if taken at the recommended doses, but they can be rather expensive.

In spite of what was said above about vitamins and supplements, you may still be persuaded by an advertisement showing a 75 year-old person cycling up a mountain path while waving his bottle of supplements. If so, do at least talk to your health care team before you buy the tablets, since they could interfere with any medication that you are already taking.

Also, don't be fooled into thinking that just because something is 'natural', that is, it exists in nature rather than having been made in a laboratory, that it is safe. Have you ever heard of poisonous mushrooms, or deadly nightshade, or ricin? These are all natural. In fact, some of the most deadly substances known to man are natural.

The Puffer fish, a delicacy in Japan, contains tetrodotoxin, a nerve poison with no known antidote. One thousandth of an ounce could kill a grown man in 20 minutes.

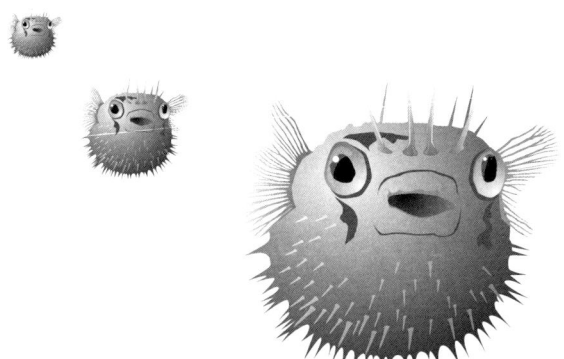

12 Some medical myths

Finally, let's consider a few medical myths. There are many of these which often find their way into the popular press. However, we shouldn't just accept these statements as fact without supporting evidence. For example, there is no evidence that we should drink at least 8 glasses of water a day. Of course, we do need a certain amount of fluid every day but we obtain this from the food and liquids that we eat and drink during our normal daily routines. If we do become short of fluid, we have a warning system – it's called getting thirsty.

Here are a few Medical Myths relevant to the topics discussed in this book.

High blood pressure causes headaches

High blood pressure is often known as the 'Silent Killer' because it usually has no symptoms. Unless it is very high it will not cause a headache.

X FALSE

Headaches can mean a brain tumour

Brain tumours are very rare. They rank 16 in the list of the commonest cancers in the UK. Headaches are very common, so it is obvious that the vast majority of headaches have nothing at all to do with brain tumours. In any case, someone with a brain tumour is likely to have other symptoms as well such as fits and changes in behaviour. So if you've just got a normal headache, don't worry

X FALSE

Sex can cause a heart attack

Having sex does involve a certain but very small amount of exertion and energy expenditure. Could this trigger a heart attack? Theoretically yes, but the increased risk is so small that it's not worth worrying about. For all practical purposes then, just enjoy.

X FALSE

People with diabetes should buy diabetic foods

Special 'diabetic' foods and drinks are available which are sweetened with substances such as lactilol. These are carbohydrates but they are not digested by the body so do not contribute to blood glucose levels. However, they can have a laxative effect. These foods are also sometimes high in fat. A healthy diet, perhaps with regular blood glucose checks, is all that is required.

X FALSE

13 Glossary

Acute Doctors separate symptoms into two categories, known as acute and chronic. An acute symptom or condition is one with a rapid onset and progression, such as acute kidney failure. This will come on suddenly, and because it involves a vital organ, needs immediate specialist attention.

Bad Cholesterol A type of cholesterol in the blood which takes it from the liver (where it is made) to various parts of the body. Also known as LDL cholesterol (Low Density Lipoprotein Cholesterol).

Blood Pressure The force exerted by the blood as it is pumped around the body by the heart, for example 140/80. The first (higher) number is the pressure as the heart contracts, and is known as the SYSTOLIC pressure. The second (lower) number is the resting pressure as the heart relaxes before the next contraction, and is known as the DIASTOLIC pressure.

Blood pressure is measured in units of millimeters of mercury (written mmHg – Hg is the chemical symbol for mercury). This refers to the height of the column of mercury in the old style machines with glass tubes.

BMI Body Mass Index A measure of whether a person is overweight or not. It is calculated by taking a person's weight in kilograms and dividing this by their height in metres squared. For example, an 80kg person who is 1.8m tall would have a BMI of 80 divided by 1.8 x 1.8 which equals 80/3.24 = 24.7. This is at the upper limit of normal.

Cholesterol A fatty substance made by the liver and also present in various foods, especially dairy foods such as cheese and eggs. It is needed by the body for the production of certain hormones and also for cell membranes, but if there is too much in the blood, it can result in fatty deposits in the blood vessels causing high blood pressure. Too much cholesterol is a risk factor for heart disease, diabetes, and stroke.

Cholesterol is measured in units of millimoles per litre (mmol/L). This is related to the number of molecules in a litre of blood. Different units are used in the USA and some other countries (milligrams per decilitre – mg/dL); this is related to the weight of the cholesterol). Unfortunately, this means that the numbers are completely different when the American units are used).

Chronic Doctors separate symptoms into two categories, known as acute and chronic. A chronic symptom or condition is one which arises gradually over a period of time, such as arthritis or diabetes.

Chronic Kidney Disease A progressive loss of kidney function which can eventually lead to complete kidney failure, necessitating dialysis or a kidney transplant. CKD can be a complication of poorly controlled diabetes.

Combination Therapy Prescribing two or more different medicines for a particular condition, each acting in a different way to attack the problem from more than one angle.

Diastolic The lower number in a blood pressure reading. It is the pressure exerted when the heart is relaxed between beats.

Glaucoma A condition in which the pressure inside the eyeball is too high. Blindness can result if this is left untreated.

Glucose Commonly referred to as 'sugar', glucose is a carbohydrate substance used by the body as a source of energy. It travels to all body tissues through the blood and its level is normally controlled by insulin. This control goes wrong in diabetes, and people with this condition may need drugs or diet and lifestyle changes to keep their glucose levels in the normal range. Glucose is measured in the blood in units of millimoles per litre (mmol/L).

Good Cholesterol A form of cholesterol in the blood which actually removes it from the circulation by taking it to the liver. Also known as HDL cholesterol (High Density Lipoprotein Cholesterol).

Hyper more than, as in hypertension meaning a blood pressure of more than normal, or hyperglycaemia meaning more sugar in the blood than normal.

Hypo under or less than, as in hypoglycaemia meaning less sugar in the blood than normal, or hypodermic meaning injecting under the skin.

Normal (Desirable) Values Studies of many thousands of healthy people have enabled doctors to establish what is considered to be normal. For example, a normal healthy adult will have a blood glucose level of between 4 and 6 units. These are known as the Normal values (or the Normal Range). Outside of these values, either higher or lower, is abnormal, and requires investigation. Note that normal values are not set in stone and may change as more medical information becomes available. It is therefore important that only the latest and most up-to-date sources are consulted. They may also vary between men and women, and between people from different ethnic backgrounds.

Omega 3 Fatty Acids Types of fatty substances needed by the body for its healthy growth and repair. Good food sources of omega 3 fatty acids are oily fish such as herring and mackerel. Capsules of omega 3 fatty acids have been used to reduce triglyceride (a type of fatty substance found in the blood although different from cholesterol) levels in people with high levels.

Risk Factors Something that increases the chance of an event happening. For example, crossing a busy road with your eyes shut is a risk factor for getting run over, and smoking cigarettes is a risk factor for getting lung cancer. Some risk factors are beyond your control and you can't do anything about them. An example would be if you had a family history of heart disease.

Statin A drug that reduces the amount of cholesterol that is made by the liver, and therefore results in a lowering of cholesterol in the blood.

Stroke An interruption to the blood supply of the brain. The effects on the patient will depend on where in the brain the stroke has occurred. There are two types of stroke. A haemorrhagic stroke is due to a bleed from a burst blood vessel, and an ischaemic stroke is due to a blockage from a blood clot.

Systolic The higher number in a blood pressure reading. It is the pressure exerted when the heart contracts.

Transient Ischaemic Attack Sometimes called a mini-stroke, this is a temporary interruption to the brain's blood flow that only lasts for a short time without any permanent damage. It is often a warning of a future full stroke and should never be ignored.

Type 1 diabetes The form of diabetes in which the pancreas is unable to produce insulin. Patients will need injections of insulin. Type 1 diabetes used to be known as Insulin-Dependent Diabetes Mellitus (IDDM).

Type 2 diabetes The form of diabetes in which the insulin produced by the pancreas is unable, for some reason, to do its job properly. Although some patients will need insulin injections, many can be treated either by diet or by tablets. Type 2 diabetes used to be known as Non-Insulin-Dependent Diabetes Mellitus (NIDDM).

Vitamins Substances that cannot be produced by the body but which are needed for healthy growth and development, and which are obtained from the diet. A lack of specific vitamins will often result in a 'deficiency disease', such as scurvy in the case of vitamin C.

Only very small amounts of vitamins are needed to stay healthy and there is no evidence that having more gives any benefits. In several cases, too much can actually cause harm, and in severe overdoses, even result in death.

Waist Circumference A simple but very effective measure of whether someone is overweight. A waist circumference is not necessarily the same as a trouser measurement. It should be taken with a tape that passes over the belly button and parallel to the ground, and be a snug fit but not pressing into the skin.

14 A few last words

It's important that you consider the advice given in this book seriously. You may know someone who was a heavy smoker all of his life and died in his sleep at 95, or someone who weighs 20 stone and is still fit and healthy well into her 80s. Such people exist but so do people who have crossed busy roads without looking and not been run over. Would you cross a road like that?

The Publishers would very much like to have your comments on this book. Did you find it helpful? Was it easy to understand? Do you have any suggestions for changes for the next edition? All comments would be gratefully received, and any ideas that are used in future editions will be rewarded with a free copy of the book.

The Publishers are also developing a website on which more information will be posted from time to time. There will also be the facility for members of the public to pose questions which will be answered by our panel of health care workers.
www.staying-alive.net

The Publishers can be contacted by email on:

info@themedicalpress.co.uk
www.staying-alive.net

15 Appendix

This is a selection of useful contact details for various organizations and websites. It is by no means a complete list but a useful starting point for further research.

Weight Loss

Weight Watchers UK Ltd
Millenium House
Ludlow Road
Maidenhead SL6 2SL
01628 418500
uk.help@weightwatchers.co.uk
www.weightwatchers.co.uk

The DASH Eating Plan
www.nhlbi.nih.gov

Slimmig World
0844 897 8000; 01773 546360
www.slimmingworld.com

High Blood Pressure and Heart Disease

British Hypertension Society
www.bhsoc.org

British Heart Foundation
14 Fitzhardinge Street
London W1H 6DH
020 7935 0185
Heart Information Line 0845 708070
www.bhf.org.uk

Blood Pressure Association
www.bpassoc.org.uk

High Blood Pressure Foundation
www.hbpf.org.uk

Heart Failure patient website
www.chfpatients.com

CASH – Consensus Action on Salt and Health
www.actiononsalt.co.uk

Heart Health Magazine
Free subscription 0870 850 5281

The American Heart Association
www.americanheart.org

Stroke

The Stroke Association
Stroke House
123-127 Whitecross Street
London EC1Y 8JJ
020 7566 0300
info@stroke.org.uk
www.stroke.org.uk

Chest, Heart & Stroke Scotland
www.chss.org.uk

Stroke Information Directory
www.stroke-info.com

Diabetes

Diabetes UK
10 Parkway
London NW1 7AA
020 7424 1000
info@diabetes.org.uk
www.diabetes.org.uk

The Diabetes Portal
www.diabetes.co.uk

South Asian Health Foundation
info@sahf.org.uk
www.sahf.org.uk

American Diabetes Association
www.diabetes.org

Diabetes Australia
www.diabetesaustralia.com

Diabetes New Zealand
www.diabetes.org.nz

Canadian Diabetes Organisation
www.diabetes.ca

Cancer

NHS Cancer Screening Programmes
The Manor House
260 Ecclesall Road South
Sheffield S11 9PS
0114 271 1060/1
www.cancerscreening.nhs.uk

European Cervical Cancer Association – ECCA
www.ecca.info

Cancer Research UK
P O Box 123
Lincoln's Inn Fields
London WC2A 3PX
020 7242 0200
cancerhelpuk@cancer.org.uk
www.cancerresearchuk.org

Action Cancer
1 Marlborough Place
Belfast BT9 6HQ
028 9066 1081
www.cancerhelp.org.uk

Smoking and Lung Disease

Action on Smoking and Health – ASH
102 Clifton Street
London EC2A 4HW
020 7739 5902
www.ash.org.uk

British Lung Foundation
78 Hatton Garden
London EC1N 8LD
020 7831 5831
www.lunguk.org

Quit
Victory House
170 Tottenham Court Road
London W1P 0HA
020 7388 5775
www.quit.org.uk

Quitline
England   0800 002200
N Ireland 02890 663281
Scotland   0800 848484
Wales   0345 697500

CancerBACUP
3 Bath Place
Rivington Street
London EC2A 3JR
0808 800 1234
www.cancerbacup.org.uk

Eye Disease

Royal College of Ophthalmologists
17 Cornwall Terrace
London NW1 4QW
020 7935 0702

The International Glaucoma Association (IGA)
Woodcote House
15 Highpoint Business Village
Henwood
Kent TN24 8DH
01233 64 81 70

Nutrition

The Food Standards Agency
tel: 020 7276 8829
helpline@foodstandards.gsi.gov.uk
www.food.gov.uk

Index

abnormal heart rhythms	32
acute	75
acute complications of diabetes	40
atrial fibrillation	32
Benecol	71
benign cancer	46
beri-beri	69
blood glucose (sugar) levels	39
blood pressure	17, 61
blood pressure measurement	18
BMI	9, 75
body mass index	9, 75
body mass index calculation	75
body mass index chart	10
bottom line summary for cancer	54
bottom line summary for cholesterol	29
bottom line summary for diabetes	43
bottom line summary for high blood pressure	23
bottom line summary for stroke	36
bottom line summary for weight loss	16
breast awareness code	50
breast cancer	49
calorie expenditure for different tasks	12
calories	11
cancer	45
cells	45
cervical cancer	50
cervical cancer vaccine	50
check list for blood pressure	19
check list for body mass index	11
check list for cholesterol	27
check list for diabetes	39
check list for heart attack risk	56, 58
check list for waist measurement	8
check list summary chart	66
cholesterol	25, 71, 76
chronic	76
chronic complications of diabetes	41
chronic kidney disease CKD	42, 76
claudication	42

colon (large bowel) cancer	48
colon cancer screening	48
combination therapy	76
commonest cancers	47
complications of diabetes	40
contact details of various health organisations	83
desirable (normal) values	77
diabetes	37, 61
diabetes complications	40
diabetes symptoms	38
diabetes treatments	40
diabetic foods	74
diastolic blood pressure	17, 76
eye tests	61
FAST campaign for stroke	34
folic acid	70
foods and calorie contents	13
glaucoma	61, 77
glossary	75
glucose (sugar)	37, 39, 77
glucose tolerance test	39
good and bad cholesterol	26, 75, 77
haemorrhagic stroke (bleed)	31
HDL cholesterol	26, 77
head injury	34
headache	73
heart attack risk	55
high blood pressure treatment	22
hyper	77
hypo	77
insulin	37
Insulin Dependent Diabetes Mellitus IDDM	79
insulin resistance	38
ischaemic stroke (clot)	31
kilojoules and joules	12
LDL cholesterol	26, 75
lipids	28
losing weight	7
lung cancer	48
lung function tests	63
malignant cancer	46
malignant melanoma	49
mammograms	49

medical myths	73
night blindness	69
Non-Insulin Dependent Diabetes Mellitus NIDDM	79
normal blood pressure	18
omega 3 fatty acids	71, 78
oral contraceptives	33
peak flow meter	63
peak flow rate	63
pellagra	69
peripheral artery disease PAD	41
peripheral vascular disease PVD	41
Pro-Activ	71
prostate cancer	51
Puffer fish	72
reducing cancer risk	48
rickets	69
risk factors	78
risk factors for high blood pressure	21
risk factors for stroke	32
salt	21
screening tests	52
scurvy	67, 69
sex and heart attacks	74
skin cancer	49
smoking	32, 53
statins	27, 78
stroke	31, 78
sun beds	49
supplements	71
systolic blood pressure	17, 79
testicular cancer	52
tetrodotoxin	72
transient ischaemic attack TIA	31, 33, 79
trouser size	7
type 1 diabetes	38, 79
type 2 diabetes	38, 79
undescended testicles	52
vitamins	67, 79
waist measurement	7, 8, 80
waist measurement, Asian and African Caribbean	8
waist measurement, desirable	8
weight loss	7
your own MOT (Medical & Optical Tests) summary	66